Cambridge Elements ☰

Elements in Emergency Neurosurgery
edited by
Nihal Gurusinghe
Lancashire Teaching Hospital NHS Trust
Peter Hutchinson
University of Cambridge, Society of British Neurological Surgeons and Royal College of Surgeons of England
Ioannis Fouyas
Royal College of Surgeons of Edinburgh
Naomi Slator
North Bristol NHS Trust
Ian Kamaly-Asl
Royal Manchester Children's Hospital
Peter Whitfield
University Hospitals Plymouth NHS Trust

MANAGEMENT OF A PATIENT WITH A VENOUS SINUS THROMBOSIS WITH OR WITHOUT AN INTRACEREBRAL HAEMATOMA

Helen Sims
North Bristol NHS Trust

James Choulerton
Royal United Hospital, Bath NHS Foundation Trust

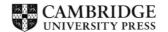

CAMBRIDGE
UNIVERSITY PRESS

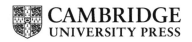

Shaftesbury Road, Cambridge CB2 8EA, United Kingdom

One Liberty Plaza, 20th Floor, New York, NY 10006, USA

477 Williamstown Road, Port Melbourne, VIC 3207, Australia

314–321, 3rd Floor, Plot 3, Splendor Forum, Jasola District Centre,
New Delhi – 110025, India

103 Penang Road, #05–06/07, Visioncrest Commercial, Singapore 238467

Cambridge University Press is part of Cambridge University Press & Assessment,
a department of the University of Cambridge.

We share the University's mission to contribute to society through the pursuit of
education, learning and research at the highest international levels of excellence.

www.cambridge.org
Information on this title: www.cambridge.org/9781009380126

DOI: 10.1017/9781009380102

© Helen Sims and James Choulerton 2025

First published 2025

A catalogue record for this publication is available from the British Library

ISBN 978-1-009-38012-6 Paperback
ISSN 2755-0656 (online)
ISSN 2755-0648 (print)

Management of a Patient with a Venous Sinus Thrombosis with or without an Intracerebral Haematoma

Elements in Emergency Neurosurgery

DOI: 10.1017/9781009380102
First published online: March 2025

Helen Sims
North Bristol NHS Trust

James Choulerton
Royal United Hospital, Bath NHS Foundation Trust

Author for correspondence: Helen Sims, helen.sims@nbt.nhs.uk

Abstract: Cerebral venous sinus thrombosis (CVST) is a serious and potentially life-threatening condition whose diagnosis is often missed or delayed due to often non-specific presentations. However, if diagnosed and managed appropriately, prognosis is generally favourable. This Element covers the common presentations and epidemiology of CVST, progressing through the approach to investigation and management of this condition in the acute, sub-acute and more chronic time frames.

Keywords: cerebral, venous, sinus, thrombosis, CVST

ISBNs: 9781009380126 (PB), 9781009380102 (OC)
ISSNs: 2755-0656 (online), 2755-0648 (print)

Contents

Epidemiology

Cerebral venous sinus thrombosis (CVST) is a serious and potentially life-threatening condition caused by partial or complete occlusion of one or more of the veins in the cerebral venous drainage system. It has a mean age of onset of 33 years, and two-thirds of cases occur in females <55 years of age (partly explained by the association with pregnancy). In those over 55, the male: female ratio is 1:1.[1]

Cerebral venous sinus thrombosis is often missed or delayed as a diagnosis due to it frequently mimicking other acute neurological conditions, with the slow growth of thrombus and recruitment of collateral supply accounting for an often slow and progressive history. However, it has a generally favourable prognosis if detected and managed early, with ~75% of patients achieving complete functional recovery. If diagnosis is delayed, around 15% of patients will die or be left dependent.[1–2]

Cerebral venous sinus thrombosis is thought to represent 0.5–1% of all unselected acute stroke admissions, with an annual recurrence rate of 2–7% and a risk of other VTE of 4–7% per year.[1–2]

About 85% of patients with CVST have at least one associated risk factor,[2] which may affect blood stasis, the vessel wall or blood composition (Virchow's triad). The most frequently identified risk factors are the following:[2–3]

- Combined oral contraceptive pill use (COCP)
- Pregnancy and the Puerperium (risk greatest with the latter)
- Genetic or Acquired prothrombotic conditions (e.g. Factor V Leiden, prothrombin gene mutation, antithrombin deficiency, Protein C and S deficiencies and antiphospholipid syndrome).

Other associated risk factors are the following:

- Infections (ears, sinuses, mouth, face and neck)
- Malignancy (accounts for ~25% of CVST in patients >55 years)
- Head injury (causing direct trauma to venous structures)
- Inflammatory diseases (e.g. systemic lupus erythematosus, Behcets, granulomatosis with polyangiitis, inflammatory bowel disease and sarcoidosis)
- Obesity
- Iron deficient anaemia
- Haematological disorders (especially myeloproliferative disorders associated with JAK2 mutations, paroxysmal nocturnal haemoglobinuria and haemoglobinopathies)
- Iatrogenic – especially during retrosigmoid or petrosal approaches to the cerebellopontine angle.

Clinical Presentation

Clinical symptoms in CVST are usually due to elevated intracranial pressure or focal brain injury from venous infarction (with or without haemorrhage). The latter process occurs because venous obstruction causes elevation in venous pressure, which leads to vasogenic oedema, decreased cerebral perfusion pressure and decreased cerebral blood flow with subsequent tissue infarction. These changes are usually initially compensated for with venous dilatation and recruitment of collateral supplies, which explains why symptoms may be insidious.

The exact clinical presentation depends on the size and location of the CVST and the extent of parenchymal injury due to venous infarction and haemorrhage.

About 90% of patients will present with a headache, which is usually non-specific in nature – with a progressive course over hours to days.[2] In 25% of cases headache may be the only clinical symptom reported.[3] Red flags for CVST in patients presenting with a new headache are persistence despite regular analgesia, symptoms of raised intracranial pressure, papilloedema and presence of risk factors for CVST.

Other common clinical symptoms and signs are as follows:[1–2]

- Focal or generalised seizures (in up to 40%)
- Focal neurology – usually not as sudden onset as with acute arterial stroke
- Reduced consciousness or coma
- Visual impairment
- Cranial nerve palsies.

Stroke-like symptoms occur in up to 40% of patients with CVST, with motor symptoms being the most common, followed by visual symptoms, aphasia and least commonly sensory disturbance.[2,4] Symptoms are often of less abrupt onset, and imaging shows infarction not discrete to a single arterial territory.

The most common location for a CVST is in the superior sagittal sinus (~60%), with the transverse sinus being the next most common location.[1]

Use of Appropriate Investigation

Urgent neuroimaging is indicated when CVST is suspected as a possible diagnosis, and maintaining a high index of suspicion is needed in order to ensure both that cases are not missed and that patients receive timely investigation. The most commonly accessible initial investigation is a non-contrast CT head scan, which is usually followed by a CT venogram (CTV).

Up to 30% of initial non-contrast CT scans may be normal; however, clot may be visible, appearing as a hyperdense triangle within the venous sinus[5–6] (Figure 1). This finding is often termed the 'dense triangle' or 'delta' sign. In

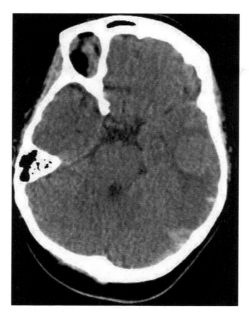

Figure 1 Acute left transverse sinus thrombosis on plain CT

addition, CT may show evidence of infarction, distinct from classical arterial infarction by appearing not to fit a single arterial territory, and also often with a prominent haemorrhagic component, being consistent with a venous infarction (Figure 2).

Either CT or MR venography can be used to confirm the presence of thrombus. The CTV is more easily accessible and rapid, meaning that it is often performed in preference to MRV. It has a sensitivity of 95% and specificity of 91% for CVST,[7] but there is the potential for false positives as a result of anatomical variations with hypoplastic sinuses and arachnoid granulations. The CTV also has low sensitivity for small thromboses and small parenchymal lesions.

Typical findings on CTV are as follows:

- Sinus or vein hyperdensity with absence of flow in thrombosed sinuses
- Empty delta sign – contrast outlines a triangular filling defect (due to thrombus) in the superior sagittal sinus, making it looks like a delta sign
- Cord sign – cord-like high attenuation within a dural venous sinus, most commonly the transverse sinus.

MRI is the most sensitive non-invasive imaging modality for detecting thrombus so long as blood sensitive sequences are performed. MR Venogram (MRV) provides time of flight and flow imaging, rather than luminal imaging like CTV. The

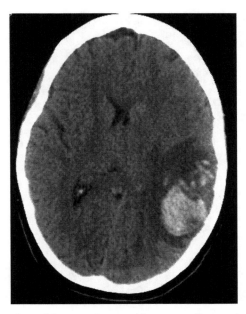

Figure 2 Flame shaped haemorrhage with surrounding oedema and venous
infarction

appearance of thrombus on MRI sequences changes over time, so while this can
help towards the ageing of the thrombus, it can also complicate interpretation.

- Up to one week: thromboses are isointense on T1 and hypointense on T2
  imaging
- At one to two weeks: Thromboses are hyperintense on T1 and T2 sequences
- At more than two weeks: Thrombosis appearance can be variable on T1 and
  T2 sequences but is hypointense on GRE and SWI imaging
- Thromboses are often hyperintense on DWI sequences
- Venous wall enhancement can often be seen.

MRI and MRV have benefits for some patients as they involve no ionising
radiation and intravenous contrast is not needed. They have much better sensitivity for detection of small parenchymal lesions and small thromboses, but are
much more time-consuming, often resulting in motion artefact as they are less
well tolerated by patients. MRI is less readily available in many places than CT
imaging and can be contraindicated in some patients, for example those with
older cardiac pacemakers.

Invasive catheter angiography is rarely needed to confirm the diagnosis of
CVST given the widespread availability of CTV and MRV, but may be indicated
where the diagnosis is unclear from initial imaging.

Ongoing Investigation

D-dimer is not indicated as a normal value does not rule out the possibility of a CVST.

In patients with a first unprovoked CVST, onward referral to haematology for further investigation is indicated and a screen for prothrombotic haematological conditions is often undertaken. It is also important to be vigilant for any suggestion of an underlying malignancy which may necessitate whole body CT imaging.

Management of CVST

Acute Management

Once a diagnosis of CVST is confirmed, treatment with therapeutic anticoagulation should start as early as possible, even if there is evidence of associated intracranial haemorrhage (e.g. into an area of venous infarction or more rarely when CVST is associated with subarachnoid haemorrhage).

Initial anticoagulation should be with parenteral heparin rather than oral anticoagulants. Parenteral administration allows for more rapid anticoagulation and although the overall strength of evidence for this approach is weak, it is a widely accepted in clinical practice across the globe.[8]

Low molecular weight heparin is the usual first line treatment and is often administered as a split dose in order to try to minimise the risk of haemorrhagic complications. Unfractionated heparin can be used in patients considered high risk of extracranial haemorrhage, with significant renal impairment (CrCl < 30 ml/min) or in those who may need rapid reversal of anticoagulation, for example those requiring neurosurgery. However, unfractionated heparin is difficult to manage accurately in any setting other than a high dependency area where regular APTT testing can be performed and results acted on promptly.

It is very important to identify and manage any underlying cause of CVST, including treatment of infection and dehydration and withdrawal of any pro-thrombotic medications such as the COCP.

Around 30% of patients present with seizure and so it is important to consider management of any seizure activity (see Woodfield and Duncan, *Management of Seizures in Neurosurgical Practice*, Elements in Emergency Neurosurgery, Cambridge University Press, 2024). There is limited evidence around the management of seizures in CVST; however, the following principles are suggested.[1]

- In those with clinical evidence of seizures, particularly where there is paren-chymal brain damage, antiepileptic treatment is appropriate.

- There is no evidence for prophylactic antiepileptic medication.
- It is important to ensure that any antiepileptic drug selected does not interact with the planned anticoagulant therapy.
- Despite a lack of evidence regarding the duration of treatment with antiepileptics in CVST, a pragmatic approach is that seizures associated with oedema, infarction or haemorrhage merit treatment for at least one year.

Seizures can also be a late complication of CVST, arising as a result of longer-term damage from prior venous infarction or haemorrhage. Decisions regarding antiepileptics should be made on an individual, case-by-case basis.

Ongoing Anticoagulation

Following on from the initial management with parenteral anticoagulation (typically around seven days), it is recommended that patients receive ongoing anticoagulation with a vitamin K antagonist aiming for an International Normalised Ratio (INR) of 2.0–3.0.

Evidence is sparse regarding the recommended length of anticoagulation for CVST and depends on factors such as individual patient risk factors balanced alongside their risk of bleeding complications.

The following are suggested approaches:[1]

- One CVST and transient risk factor (e.g. dehydration, infection, COCP, surgery and trauma)

  o Three to six months anticoagulation

- One CVST of unknown cause

  o 6–12 months anticoagulation

- Two or more CVSTs (or one CVST and ongoing risk factors indicating high thrombotic risk)

  o Lifelong.

There is currently no clear evidence to support the use of Direct Oral Anti-Coagulants (DOACs) versus warfarin for the treatment of CVST; however, a recent systematic review indicated similar outcomes from limited data whilst highlighting the need for further rigorous trials in this area.[9] In our experience, some physicians pragmatically elect to prescribe DOACs based on their license for the treatment of peripheral VTE, ease of administration and the lower risk of intracranial bleeding compared to warfarin (Figure 3).

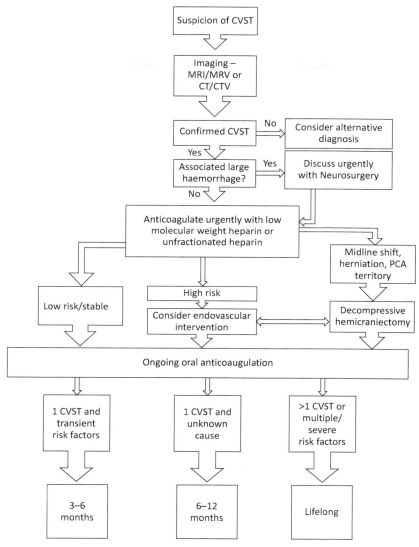

Figure 3 Guidelines

Endovascular Treatment

Evidence for the efficacy of endovascular thrombolysis and thrombectomy is limited despite a reported recanalisation rate of up to 75%.[10]
There are mainly only small case series assessing clinical effectiveness
with only one randomised trial which showed no clear benefit for endovascular treatment over standard medical care.[11] In our experience, endovascular therapies are only ever considered if there is a contraindication

to anticoagulation or clinical deterioration or progression despite therapeutic anticoagulation.

Neurosurgery

Management of Raised Intracranial Pressure (ICP)

Patients at high risk of raised intracranial pressure, including those with evidence of vasogenic oedema, significant cerebral infarction and extensive intracranial haemorrhagic, should ideally be managed in a high dependency or critical care setting, because they are at highest risk of significant brain injury and death.

Strategies for managing raised intracranial pressure include the following:

- Mannitol can be used for osmotic therapy. There is no evidence for the use of acetazolamide
- Hyperventilation aiming for PCO2 3–3.5
- Head elevation
- Therapeutic lumbar puncture (contraindicated in patients with large lesions at risk of herniation).

There is no evidence for the routine use of acetazolamide, corticosteroids or ventricular shunting in managing elevated intracranial pressure.

If there is evidence of midline shift or herniation on brain imaging, then medical therapy is unlikely to suffice and patients should be considered for decompressive hemicraniectomy.

Decompressive Craniotomy

Decompressive craniotomy is a procedure intended to mitigate the effects of raised ICP in those patients with brain lesions causing mass effect or clinical deterioration. It allows swollen brain to expand and potential recruitment of collateral venous drainage vessels which can both help reduce pressure. There is no randomised controlled trial (RCT) data for decompressive craniotomy in CVST but observational data suggest that it can be a life-saving treatment with favourable outcomes reported in over half of patients, even in some with clinically concerning features such as fixed dilated pupils.[12]

Complications and Prognosis

Around 75% of patients with CVST achieve a favourable outcome, with the rest either dying or being left dependent. Risk factors for worse outcomes include older age, male sex, confusion or coma, haemorrhage on initial CT, deep vein involvement, central nervous system infection and cancer.[2] In those patients who achieve a good recovery, there may be persisting deficits affecting cognition, fatigue, depression or anxiety; however, the incidence of these are not fully known, and are likely to be under-reported and under-diagnosed. The risk of recurrent CVST is fortunately reasonably low, quoted at around 2–7% per year.[1]

Dural Arteriovenous Fistulas (dAVF)

Dural arteriovenous fistulas are a rare complication of CVST and the relationship between the two and how they occur is not fully understood. It is thought that progressive narrowing and occlusion of the large deep venous system, and the recruitment of collateral supply that can ensue, causes abnormal connections to form between the arterial and venous system in the dura mater. They can be symptomatic with headache, symptoms and signs of raised ICP, or with haemorrhagic complications, or can be asymptomatic. It is important to be aware of the possibility of the formation of dAVFs as early identification allows for early treatment. Treatment options involve endovascular coiling, stereotactic radiotherapy and surgery (see Kirollos and Kirollos, *Spontaneous Intracranial Haemorrhage Caused by a Non-aneurysmal Brain Vascular Malformation*, Elements in Emergency Neurosurgery, Cambridge University Press, forthcoming).

Vaccine-Induced Thrombotic Thrombocytopenia (VITT)

Vaccine-induced thrombotic thrombocytopenia has recently been identified as a rare complication of COVID-19 vaccinations. This condition can cause both arterial and venous thromboses, with CVST being the most common presentation. Compared to non-VITT patients, those with VITT-associated CVST have more extensive thrombosis, increased rates of extracranial thrombosis and higher rates of multiple intracerebral haemorrhages.[13] VITT-associated CVST appears to have higher mortality of up to 40%[14] and increased dependency rates too; around half of these patients have modified rankin scores (mRS) of 3–6 compared with the 15% in those with non-VITT CVST.[13]

Vaccine-induced thrombotic thrombocytopenia has been reported with two adenovirus vector COVID-19 vaccines (ChAdOx1 and Ad.26.COV2.S) and typically presents 7–10 days after administration of the first vaccine dose.

There have been some reports of thrombocytopenia following vaccination with mRNA vaccines (mRNA-1273 and BNT162b2), but this is more commonly associated with purpura and mucosal bleeding rather than thrombotic complications such as CVST.

To make a definitive diagnosis of VITT, the following five criteria must be met:[15]

1. COVID vaccine 4–42 days prior to symptom onset
2. Any venous or arterial thrombosis (often cerebral or abdominal)
3. Thrombocytopenia (platelet count $< 150 \times 10^9$/L)
4. Positive PF4 'HIT' (heparin-induced thrombocytopenia) ELISA
5. Markedly elevated D-dimer (>four times upper limit of normal).

Differential diagnoses for VITT include the following:

- Thrombosis associated with disseminated malignancy
- Disseminated intravascular coagulation
- Heparin-induced thrombocytopenia
- Thrombotic thrombocytopenic purpura
- Paroxysmal nocturnal haemoglobinuria
- Acute/chronic liver disease.

Management of VITT broadly follows recommendations for treating heparin-induced thrombocytopaenia (HIT), given the clinical similarities between the two clinical conditions.[16] Accordingly, patients with VITT-associated thrombosis should not be anticoagulated using heparin-based anticoagulants, and instead should receive anticoagulants such as fondaparinux, argobatran or direct oral anticoagulants (DOACs). If the latter agents are used, then at least five days of parenteral anticoagulation should be given prior to starting a DOAC.

Based on evidence of response in HIT, and given the underlying immunological basis of the condition, treatment with Intravenous Immunoglobulins (IVIg) 1 g/kg body weight daily for two days is needed alongside anticoagulation.[16] If there is poor response to IVIg, then IV corticosteroids (e.g. Methylprednisolone) and plasma exchange with fresh frozen plasma can be pragmatically tried as the second line treatment. Eculizumab has shown some benefit in patients who have not responded to a second dose of IVIg, but evidence and data surrounding these treatments is sparse in this new condition with relatively small numbers.[15]

Clinical Vignette

A 45-year-old female presents to the Emergency Department with three- to four-day long history of headache and dizziness, followed by development of slurred speech, agitation and disorientation. She had ingested a large amount of alcohol on the day of admission and had been vomiting for several hours.

On review she had evidence of expressive and receptive aphasia and was agitated. She had GCS 12/15 (E3, V4, M5). There was no obvious focal weakness, but examination was limited due to her agitation. She was initially given Dexamethasone and Aciclovir to treat a suspected encephalitis, but when the CT head was done it showed a large left temporoparietal haematoma with surrounding low density and moderate mass effect and midline shift.

She returned to scan for a CTV, which showed extensive thrombus within the left transverse and sigmoid sinus. She was started on treatment dose dalteparin. As her agitation improved, it became evident that she also had a right-sided homonymous hemianopia.

A thrombophilia screen was sent, which was all negative (immunoglobulins, ANCA, ACLA, ANA, Hep 2, plasma viscosity, lupus anticoagulant). She had a CT chest/abdomen/pelvis which showed no evidence of underlying malignancy or other explanation for her CVST.

On Haematology advice she was changed to Apixaban on discharge, and was followed up in the anticoagulation clinic. No underlying cause of her CVST could be found and it was classified as a spontaneous CVST. Her anticoagulation was stopped at six months, with evidence showing no benefit of continuing lifelong in a first spontaneous CVST, with recurrence risk being 2.8%.

References

1. Ulivi L, Squitieri M, Cohen H, Cowley P, Werring DJ. Cerebral venous thrombosis: A practical guide. Pract Neurol. October 2020; 20(5): 356–367. https://doi.org/10.1136/practneurol-2019-002415. PMID: 32958591.

2. Ferro JM, Canhão P, Stam J, Bousser MG, Barinagarrementeria F ; ISCVT Investigators. Prognosis of cerebral vein and dural sinus thrombosis: Results of the International Study on Cerebral Vein and Dural Sinus Thrombosis (ISCVT). Stroke. March 2004; 35(3): 664–670. https://doi.org/10.1161/01.STR.0000117571.76197.26. Epub 19 February 2004. PMID: 14976332.

3. Saposnik G, Barinagarrementeria F, Brown R, et al. Diagnosis and management of cerebral venous thrombosis. Stroke. April 2011; 42(4): 1158–1192. https://doi.org/10.1161/STR/0b013e31820a8364. PMID: 21293023.

4. Duman T, Uluduz D, Midi I, Orken DN, Aluclu U. A multicenter study of 1144 patients with cerebral venous thrombosis the VENOST study. J Stroke Cerebrovas Dis. August 2017; 26(8): 1848–1857. https://doi.org/10.1016/jstrokecerebrovasdis.2017.04.020. PMID: 28583818.

5. Bousser MG, Ferro J. Cerebral venous thrombosis: An update. Lancet Neurol. February 2007; 6(2): 162–170. https://doi.org/10.1016/S1474-4422(07)70029-7. PMID: 17239803.

6. Garetier M, Rousset J, Pearson E, et al. Value of spontaneous hyperdensity of cerebral venous thrombosis on helical CT. Acta Radiol. December 2014; 55(10): 1245–1252. https://doi.org/10.1177/0284185113513977. PMID: 24277885.

7. Wetzel SG, Kirsch E, Stock KW, et al. Cerebral veins: Comparative study of CT venography with intraarterial digital subtraction angiography. Am J Neuroradiol. February 1999; 20(2): 249–255. PMID 10094346. PMCID: PMC7056122.

8. Coutinho J. de Bruijn SFTM, deVeber G, Stam J. Anticoagulation for cerebral venous sinus thrombosis. Cochrane Database Syst Rev. August 2011; 2011(8): CD002005. https://doi.org/10.1002/14651858.CD002005.pub2. PMID: 21833941. PMCID: PMC7065450.

9. Bose G, Graveline J, Yogendrakumar V, et al. Direct oral anticoagulants in treatment of cerebral venous thrombosis: A systematic review. BMJ Open. February 2021; 11(2): e040212. https://doi.org/10.1136/bmjopen-2020-040212. PMID: 335937766. PMCID: PMC7888326.

10. Siddiqui FM, Dandapat S, Banerjee C, et al. Mechanical thrombectomy in cerebral venous thrombosis: Systematic review of 185 cases. Stroke. May

2015; 46(5): 1263–1268. https://doi.org/10.1161/STROKEAHA.114.007465. Epub 21 April 2015. PMID: 25899238.

11. Coutinho JM, Zuurbier SM, Bousser M, et al. Effect of endovascular treatment with medical management vs standard care on severe cerebral venous thrombosis: The TO-ACT randomized clinical trial. JAMA Neurol. 2020; 77(8): 966–973. https://doi.org/10.1001/jamaneurol.2020.1022.

12. Ferro JM, Crassard I, Coutinho JM, et al.; Second International Study on Cerebral Vein and Dural Sinus Thrombosis (ISCVT 2) Investigators. Decompressive surgery in cerebrovenous thrombosis: A multicenter registry and a systematic review of individual patient data. Stroke. October 2011; 42(10): 2825–2831. https://doi.org/10.1161/STROKEAHA.111.615393. Epub 28 July 2011. PMID: 21799156.

13. Perry RJ, Tamborska A, Singh B, et al.; CVT after Immunisation against COVID-19 (CAIAC) collaborators. Cerebral venous thrombosis after vaccination against COVID-19 in the UK: A multicentre cohort study. Lancet. 25 September 2021; 398(10306): 1147–1156. https://doi.org/10.1016/S0140-6736(21)01608-1. Epub 6 August 2021. PMID: 34370972; PMCID: PMC8346241.

14. Jaiswal V, Nepal G, Dijamco P, et al. Cerebral venous sinus thrombosis following COVID-19 vaccination: A systematic review. J Prim Care Community Health. January–December 2022; 13: 21501319221074450. https://doi.org/10.1177/21501319221074450. PMID: 35142234; PMCID: PMC8841914.

15. Bussel JB, Connors JM, Cines DB, et al. Thrombosis with thrombocytopenia syndrome (also termed Vaccine-induced Thrombotic Thrombocytopenia). American Society of Hematology. Accessed 2 April 2023. www.hematology.org:443/covid-19/vaccine-induced-immunethrombotic-thrombocytopenia.

16. Furie KL, Cushman M, Elkind MSV, Lyden PD, Saposnik G. Diagnosis and management of cerebral venous sinus thrombosis with vaccine-induced immune thrombotic thrombocytopenia. Stroke. 2021; 52(7): 2478–2482. https://doi.org/10.1161/STROKEAHA.121.035564.

Cambridge Elements ☰

Emergency Neurosurgery

Nihal Gurusinghe
Lancashire Teaching Hospital NHS Trust

Professor Nihal Gurusinghe is a Consultant Neurosurgeon at the Lancashire Teaching Hospitals NHS Trust. He is on the Executive Council of the Society of British Neurological Surgeons as the Lead for NICE (National Institute for Health and Care Excellence) guidelines relating to neurosurgical practice. He is also an examiner for the UK and International FRCS examinations in Neurosurgery.

Peter Hutchinson
University of Cambridge, Society of British Neurological Surgeons and Royal College of Surgeons of England

Peter Hutchinson BSc MBBS FFSEM FRCS(SN) PhD FMedSci is Professor of Neurosurgery and Head of the Division of Academic Neurosurgery at the University of=Cambridge, and Honorary Consultant Neurosurgeon at Addenbrooke's Hospital. He is Director of Clinical Research at the Royal College of Surgeons of England and Meetings Secretary of the Society of British Neurological Surgeons.

Ioannis Fouyas
Royal College of Surgeons of Edinburgh

Ioannis Fouyas is a Consultant Neurosurgeon in Edinburgh. His clinical interests focus on the treatment of complex cerebrovascular and skull base pathologies. His academic endeavours concentrate in the field of cerebrovascular pathophysiology. His passion is technical surgical training, fulfilled in collaboration with the Royal College of Surgeons of Edinburgh. Finally, he pursues Undergraduate Neuroscience teaching, with a particular focus on functional Neuroanatomy.

Naomi Slator
North Bristol NHS Trust

Naomi Slator FRCS (SN) is a Consultant Spinal Neurosurgeon based at North Bristol NHS Trust. She has a specialist interest in Complex Spine alongside Cranial and Spinal Trauma. She completed her neurosurgical training in Birmingham and a six-month Fellowship in CSF and Trauma (2019). She then went on to complete her Spinal Fellowship in Leeds (2020) before moving to the southwest to take up her consultant post.

Ian Kamaly-Asl
Royal Manchester Children's Hospital

Ian Kamaly-Asl is a full time paediatric neurosurgeon and Honorary Chair at Royal Manchester Children's Hospital. He trained in North Western Deanery with fellowships at Boston Children's Hospital and Sick Kids in Toronto. Ian is a member of council of The Royal College of Surgeons of England and The SBNS where he is lead for mentoring and tackling oppressive behaviours.

Peter Whitfield

University Hospitals Plymouth NHS Trust

Professor Peter Whitfield is a Consultant Neurosurgeon at the South West Neurosurgical Centre, University Hospitals Plymouth NHS Trust. His clinical interests include vascular neurosurgery, neuro oncology and trauma. He has held many roles in postgraduate neurosurgical education and is President of the Society of British Neurological Surgeons. Peter has published widely, and is passionate about education, training and the promotion of clinical research.

About the Series

Elements in Emergency Neurosurgery is intended for trainees and practitioners in Neurosurgery and Emergency Medicine as well as allied specialties all over the world. Authored by international experts, this series provides core knowledge, common clinical pathways and recommendations on the management of acute conditions of the brain and spine.

Cambridge Elements ≣

Emergency Neurosurgery

Elements in the Series

A full series listing is available at: www.cambridge.org/EEMN

Printed in the United States
by Baker & Taylor Publisher Services